Yoga

The 30 Greatest Yoga Poses For Beginners

Table of Contents

Introduction

Yoga is a very ancient practice, whose exact origin is yet to be traced. While some claim its presence has been around for more than 5000 years, there are others who feel that yoga had been practiced by people who lived more than 10,000 years ago. This beautiful form of exercise that originated in India is now being practiced across the globe, of course, with countless variations in the style of practice.

Yet, the core form is still Hatha Yoga, which in fact is a mild, yet strong set of postures, breathing techniques, Mudras or gestures, meditations, and Bandhas [energy locks]. Ashtanga Yoga, Iyengar Yoga, Power Yoga, Bikram Yoga, Sivananda Yoga, Kundalini Yoga – there are countless variants, including the latest ones like aerial yoga and aqua yoga, from which you can choose a style that suits your needs.

While yoga, indeed, helps in curing various physical ailments, it primarily deals with managing your mind. It teaches you the numerous ways you can improve and enhance your mental clarity and balance. When your mind is clear, your physical health is always balanced.

Yoga teaches you to restore this lost natural balance through its postures, breathing techniques, and meditation practice. The concepts of yoga looks simple, but it is like a treasure hunt.

"Yoga does not remove us from the reality or responsibilities of everyday life but rather places our feet firmly and resolutely in the practical ground of experience. We don't transcend our lives; we return to the life we left behind in the hopes of something better," says Donna Farhi, a renowned yoga teacher.

So, are you ready for the treasure hunt?

Chapter 1

Why should you practice yoga?

Well, the first answer that pops out of the mouth of many yoga practitioners is –"Better health." According to the late yoga guru B.K.S. Iyengar, *"Healthy plants and trees yield abundant flowers and fruits. Similarly, from a healthy person, smiles and happiness shine forth like the rays of the sun."*

While this is 100% true, what we forget is that yoga works on your body-mind connection. *"I have been a seeker and I still am, but I stopped asking the books and the stars. I started listening to the teaching of my Soul."*

Thus goes the words of Jalāl ad-Dīn Muhammad Rūmī, the world famous poet and scholar. And, if you take a close look at these simple words, you will identify that yoga is the best and perhaps, the most natural way to start listening to your Soul. Yes, when you start listening to your mind, your physical health will be restored to its natural state.

Countless researches conducted on the impact of yoga pertaining to health prove that regular practice of yoga could help manage or control a wide array of health conditions.

Yoga

- ➢ Boosts your flexibility, strength, structural alignment, muscle tone, and stamina

- ➢ Eases tension, stress, nervousness, and anxiety

- ➢ Boosts self-confidence and self-esteem

- ➢ Enhances creativity, memory, focus, and concentration

- ➢ Helps in shedding the excess weight

- ➢ Improves circulation

- ➢ Improves the functioning of digestive system

- ➢ Stimulates your immune system

- ➢ Improves mental steadiness

- ➢ Inculcates a sense of peace, calm, and well-being

Now that you know why you should do yoga, can we move on to take a look at how yoga helps in healing your body and mind?

Chapter 2

Yoga as a cure for body and mind 'dis-eases'

Life, today, is complex, clogged with stress, tension, and anxiety. No one has time for oneself. It is always a hectic life which does not have any meaning. The result – your tummy starts popping out, your hips turn stiff, your wrists fight to move as it should, and not to forget the nagging headache.

And, we rush to the doctors and pop in some pills to ease these conditions. There is a shortcut for every ailment now. There are countless tricks out there that seem to be working on everyone but not on you, right? Well, it is now time to take a break from all those so-called 'magic' solutions.

Try yoga! Yoga encourages you to travel to a destination where there is nothing, except good and purity. No one is bad or nothing is wrong here. And, don't worry about twisting and tweaking your body into those pretzel-like postures. Ok, I do agree that yoga does have some complicated postures, but those are meant for the advanced practitioners, which you could also become with regular and dedicated practice. Till then, take it easy. All you need to do yoga is to know how to inhale and exhale consciously.

Said that, we will now just briefly take a few steps down to see how yoga helps in healing your body and mind.

Yoga and weight loss

Asanas, or the physical postures, we practice in Yoga work on various body systems, enticing and coaxing them to return to their actual functional mode. When your circulation improves, your digestion enhances. When your digestion is on track, your toxins are eliminated properly and naturally. A toxin-free body is metabolically active, which in turn, burns the excess calories stored. When the stored-up fat is used to produce energy, you will find yourself fitting into smaller sizes.

On a mental level, it eases the stress and helps you become more aware of what you eat. You will find yourself eating less. When you eat less, as I said, the body starts using up the reserves, promoting weight loss. Bonus – your cortisol levels come down, which is beneficial for shedding the excess pounds.

Yoga for stress and anxiety

Various yoga postures when practiced along with a breathing and meditation sequence teaches you to regulate your breath and relax your mind and body, when you come under the attack of stress and anxiety. These techniques flood all the body parts and brain with a fresh dose of blood, oxygen, and nutrients, setting the stage for overall peace and relaxation.

Yoga and self-esteem

Yoga makes you aware of your strengths and limitations. It strengthens your mind, enabling you to think and act better during crises. It corrects your posture, which quite often gets hampered due to lack of confidence and low self-esteem.

Talking in terms of Chakras or the energy centers of the body, various yoga postures help in activating the Manipura or Solar Plexus chakra, which is the center of self-esteem. A balanced Solar Plexus is what makes you accept your true self unconditionally.

So, are you ready to uncover the treasures that are hidden within you?

Fasten your seat belts…. And, here we go…

Chapter 3

30 Minute Fat Burning Yoga

"Yoga is about balance, both mind and body, as well as increasing self-awareness, with by-products of better strength and flexibility," says M.E. Dahkid, the author of *"Yoga: The Essential Guide: How to Master Weight Loss, Stress Reduction and Find Inner Peace."*

The sequence comprises of a couple of warm-up exercises to oxygenate your body and prepare it for the postures that follow. There are around 13 postures, which you need to practice at least two rounds so as to boost your metabolic rate. The sequence ends with Corpse Pose that would help you summarize the whole practice and reap the benefits.

Warming Up with Breathing & Stretches

1. Sit down in a comfortable seated position, keeping the spine erect, neck and shoulders relaxed, palms resting on

the knees with the tips of index finger and thumb touching each other. Close your eyes.

2. Inhale and expand your belly. Exhale and pull your navel in and close to your spine.

3. Feel the air moving in and out of the belly, energizing your core and body for the practice.

4. Do 5 such rounds.

5. At the end of 5 rounds, lift your legs off the mat, keeping the knees straight, and allow it to come parallel to the floor.

6. Extend your hands parallel to your legs. Keep the spine nice and long and ensure that your sit bones are resting on the mat. Engage the abdominal muscles and buttocks firmly.

7. Inhale and stretch backward and rolling your shoulders back. Keep the neck and face relaxed. Stretch back until you are a couple of inches of the floor and your body resembles a low boat.

8. Exhale and lift your torso making 45 degree angle with the mat. Your body will resemble a high boat. As you come back to this position, feel the core being pulled in towards the spine.

9. Do 10 rounds.

10. As you exhale at the end of the 10th round, place your legs on the mat, keeping the knees bent.

11. Hug your knees with your hands.

12. Inhale and stretch back on the mat, holding the knees. Exhale and come back to starting position.

13. Do 5 such rounds.

14. At the end of the 5th round, place your palms on either sides of the feet and walk your feet backward. Push your hips to the ceiling and heels to the floor.

15. Inhale and as you exhale, jump or walk in between the palms, keeping your head down and close to the shin.

16. Inhale, sweep your arms over your head, and lift your torso to take a subtle backbend.

17. Exhale and join your palms at heart center.

18. Separate your feet and keep your hands away from the body. Close your eyes and take 5 deep breaths to prepare yourself for the sequence.

20-Minute Weight Loss Sequence

The sequence starts and ends with Tadasana.

1. Tadasana – Samsthithi or Equilibrium Pose

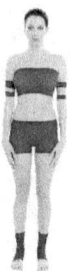

This pose helps to concentrate your thoughts and create an awareness about your body.

How to do:

1. Stand on the front of the mat, feet touching each other and firmly placed into the mat.

2. Keep your spine erect, hands joined at your heart center. Keep the neck and head relaxed.

2. Utkatasana – Chair Pose

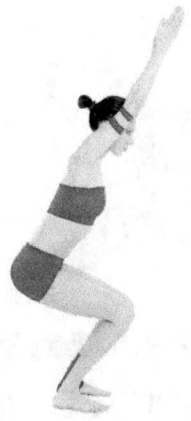

Tone your legs and sculpt your abs while strengthening your spine and back with this pose.

How to do:

1. Inhale, and bend your knees until fingertips touch the mat.

2. Sweep your hands over your head and join your palms.

3. Push your hips back like you are sitting on a chair and adjust the knees in such a way that it is stacked over the ankles.

4. Pull your navel in and close to the spine.

5. Hold the posture for 5 deep breaths.

3. Parivrtta Parsvakonasana - Revolved Side Angle Pose

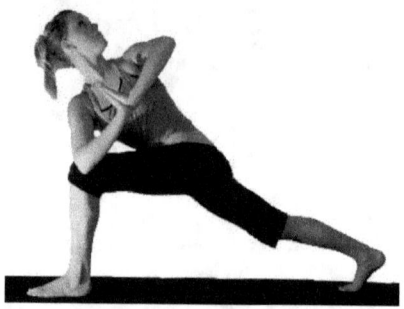

This is a simple twist that works towards improving your digestion. It also tones your torso.

How to do:

1. Inhale and stretch your right leg backward. Keep the toes tucked.

2. Exhale, twist to your left, and bring your arms outside of your left knee, keeping the palms joined.

3. Hold the posture for 5 deep breaths.

4. Anjaneyasana – Lunge Pose

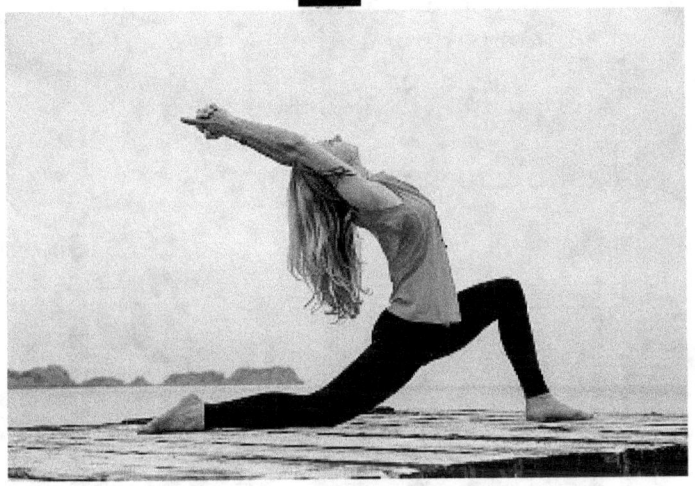

It strengthens and tones your thighs and quadriceps, while toning your abdominal muscles and back.

How to do:

1. On the final exhalation of Revolved Side Angle Pose, place the right knee down, extending the toes backward.

2. Inhale and sweep your hands up and over your head, joining your palms. Push the hips squared and down and close to the mat. Keep the left knee stacked over the ankle.

3. Take a gentle backbend, tilting your head back to gaze at the fingertips. If you have high blood pressure, dizziness

or neck issue, keep your head and neck straight, fixing your gaze at a point in front of you.

4. Hold for 5 deep breaths.

5. Kumbhakasana – Plank Pose

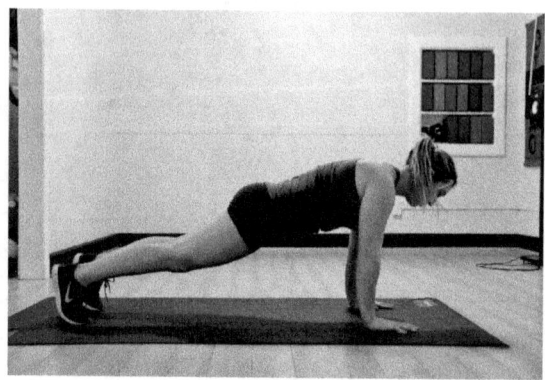

Tone your core, legs, and arms with this wonderful arm balance.

1. **How to do:**

1. With the final exhalation in the Lunge, lift your right knee off the mat, tucking the toes.

2. Inhale and place your left leg back and close to the right leg, keeping the toes tucked.

3. Align the wrists in such a way that they are stacked under the shoulders. Spread the fingers wide and strong.

4. Engage your core, glutes, and quadriceps, and roll back the shoulders.

5. Gaze forward and hold the posture for 5 deep breaths.

6. Vasisthasana – Side Plank Pose

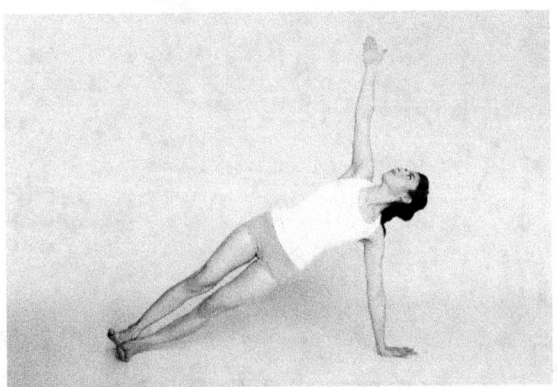

It tones and strengthens your arms, belly, and legs. It is also beneficial to improve your balance and awareness.

How to do:

1. Inhale and twist to your right, stacking your right feet over the left.

2. Exhale and lift the right arm up. Hold the pose for 2 deep breaths.

3. At the end of second exhalation, come back to the Plank pose.

4. Inhale and twist to your left, stacking your left feet over the right.

5. Exhale and lift the left arm up. Hold the pose for 2 deep breaths.

6. At the end of second exhalation, come back to the Plank Pose.

7. Repeat 5 times on each side.

7. Kumbhakasana

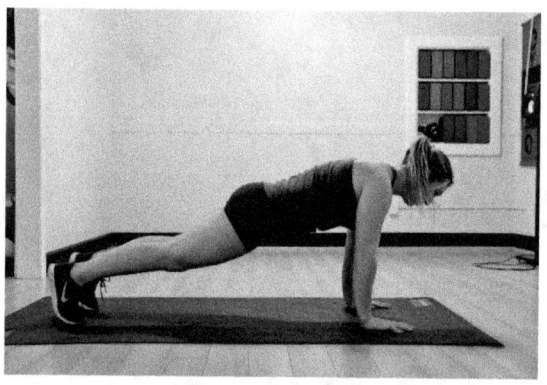

At the end of the final round, come back to the Plank Pose.

8. Bhujangasana – Cobra Pose

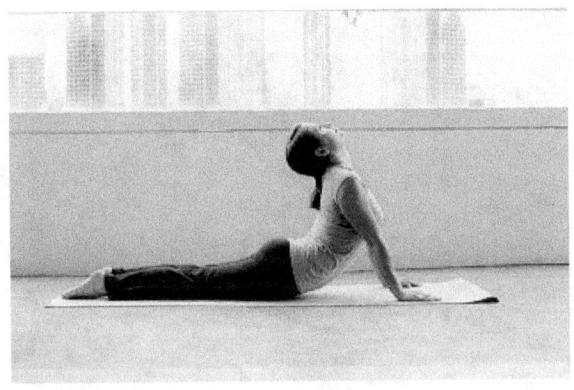

A simple backbend, it heals and strengthens your back muscles.

How to do:

1. From the Plank, exhale and lie down on the mat on your tummy, keeping the elbows bent and off the floor, yet close to your body. Keep the toes extended backward.

2. Inhale, push the palms firmly into the mat, and lift your head and torso, till your navel off the mat, and bend backward gently.

3. Hold the posture, straightening the elbows, and gazing up for 5 deep breaths.

9. Adho Mukha Svanasana – Downward Facing Dog Pose

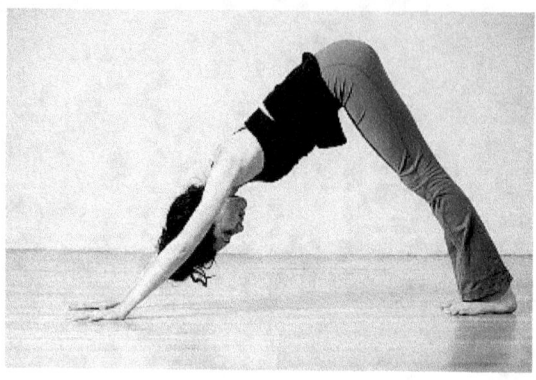

It stretches your arms and legs and promotes relaxation and peace.

How to do:

1. On the final exhalation in the Cobra pose, tuck your toes and lift your body off the floor.

2. Push your pelvis and hips towards the ceiling, heels move towards the mat.

3. Spread the palms wide and stack the wrists under the shoulders, your head coming closer to the mat, in between the elbows.

4. Hold the posture, engaging the core muscles for 5 deep breaths.

10. Uttanasana – Standing Forward Fold

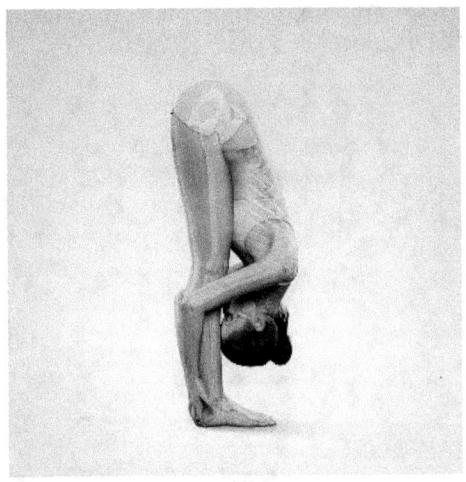

This posture works on your abdomen and helps in improving the flexibility of your hamstrings. A good stress-buster, it helps in toning your back and thighs also.

How to do:

1. With the final exhalation in Downward facing dog pose, walk or jump in between your palms, and fold forward, allowing your head to come close to the feet.

2. Keep your knees bent, if you have a bad back or knee injury. Keep the palms wherever they are, either flat or on the fingertips.

3. Hold the posture for 5 deep breaths.

11. Utkatasana – Chair Pose

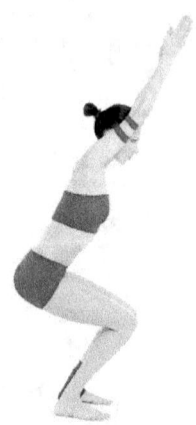

How to do:

1. Inhale and bend your knees, pushing the hips back like you are sitting on a chair, and stacking the knees over the ankles.

2. Exhale and sweep your hands over your head, joining the palms.

3. Hold the posture for 5 deep breaths.

12. Ardha Chakrasana – Half Wheel Pose

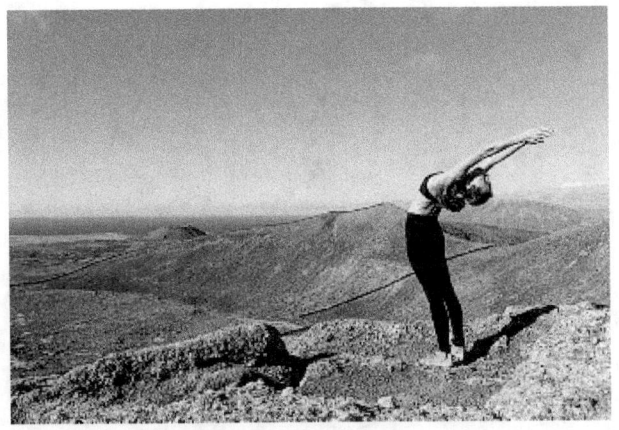

This is a backbend which helps in easing the tension experienced by the body and strengthens your core.

How to do:

1. Inhale and straighten your knees and torso.

2. Take a gentle backbend, sweeping your arms over your head, joining the palms.

3. Hold the posture for 5 deep breaths.

13. Tadasana – Equilibrium Pose

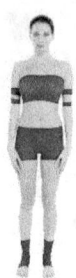

How to do:

1. Exhale and release your hands on either sides of the body.

2. Bring your body to a neutral state, keeping the spine erect, head and neck relaxed.

What to do next?

This makes only half of one round of the sequence. Take 5 deep breaths before you move into the other half.

Repeat the sequence once more, changing sides to left in the following postures.

➤ Parivrtta Parsvakonasana

➢ Anjaneyasana

While doing Side Plank, do it on the left side first.

Do the sequence one more time, repeating on either sides for better results, pausing for 5 deep breaths between repetitions.

Wind Up With Savasana

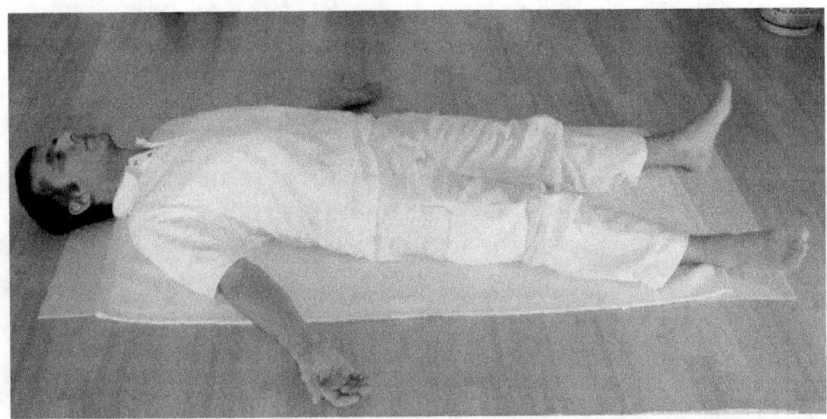

Winding up after a strenuous routine is essential to allow your body and mind to come back to its normal state. Savasana, or Corpse Pose, is a classical restorative pose that allow you to revisit your practice mentally and gather the learning.

How to do:

1. Lie down on the mat on your back.

2. Separate your legs wider than your hips, allowing the feet to fall to the sides naturally.

3. Keep your hands about 12 inches away from the body to allow the armpits to breathe.

4. Tuck your chin slightly in to give space for your armpits.

5. Close your eyes and relax, breathing deeply.

6. Let abdomen rise as you inhale and fall as you exhale.

7. Revisit your practice mentally, without any judgment, and witness it to gather your learning.

8. Once you feel you are ready, gently move your toes and fingers. Turn your head from side to side.

9. Inhale and lift your hands over your head.

10. Retain the breath and stretch your entire body.

11. Exhale, roll to your right, and sit down in any comfortable posture, keeping the eyes closed.

12. Rub your palms to generate heat.

13. Place your palms on the eyes and slowly open the eyes to the light.

Start practicing this 30 minute session right away and let the excess pounds melt away!

Chapter 4

30 Minutes to Bid Goodbye To Stress & Anxiety

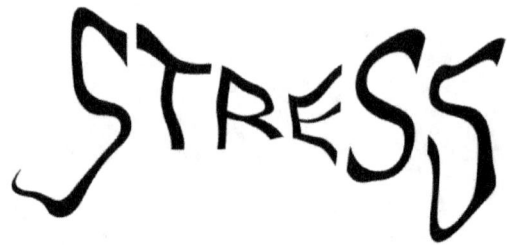

We all experience anxiety at some point in our lives. Stress, as we all know, is good to a certain extent as it helps you to showcase better performance. But, in the present era, all are plagued by chronic stress that deteriorates the quality of life as a whole.

If you feel that anxiety and stress will not affect your physical well-being, then it is time to re-think your approach. Countless studies conducted on the negative impacts of stress prove that it is one of the deadliest enemies mankind is combating. The effects of stress and continuous anxiety leads to various lethal health conditions, including obesity, hypertension, diabetes, fertility issues, cardiovascular conditions, atherosclerosis, and erectile dysfunction, to name a few.

"Yoga has a sly, clever way of short circuiting the mental patterns that cause anxiety," says Baxter Bell.

It is now time to take action. Make this 20 minute routine a part of your life and you will soon notice the changes…

Warm Up with Breathing Exercises

"When the breath wanders the mind also is unsteady. But when the breath is calmed the mind too will be still, and the yogi achieves long life. Therefore, one should learn to control the breath," says Hatha Yoga Pradipika.

And, that is why breathing is the key to busting stress and anxiety. The practice outlined below is known as the ***Breath of Fire***. It involves active inhalations and exhalations of equal frequencies with stomach moving in and out with in and out breaths.

How to do:

1. Sit down in a comfortable seated posture, keeping your spine erect and palms resting on your knees. Allow the tips of the index and thumb fingers to be in contact.

2. Take 5 rounds of deep inhalations and exhalations.

3. Allow your abdominal muscles to relax. Close your eyes.

4. Now start to breathe fast through your nose, keeping the length of the inhalations and exhalations equal. You will feel as if you are sniffing rapidly.

5. Ensure that the breath is naturally shallow.

6. Do 30 strokes at a comfortable speed.

7. Once you complete 30 strokes, pause for 3 rounds of natural breathing and repeat again.

Practice 3 to 5 rounds, pausing for 3 rounds of natural breathing between repetitions. This will take around 5 minutes.

Once you complete the Breath of Fire Pranayama, allow your body to settle down. Make conscious efforts to bring down the pace of your heart beat to its normal rate. Once you are ready, proceed to the sequence of postures.

15 Minute Stress Busting Sequence

1. Marjaryasana - Bitilasana Vinyasa – Cat-Cow Flow

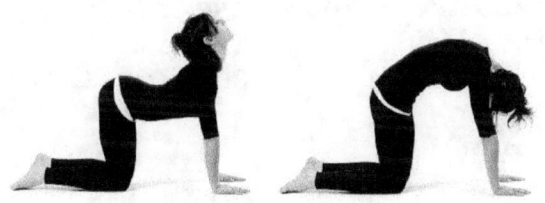

This helps in relaxing the spine and your entire body, thereby plummeting the rising cortisol levels and putting you at ease.

How to do:

1. Come on all your fours, wrists stacked under the shoulders and knees under the hips.

2. Spread your fingers wide, pushing the palms into the mat. Keep the toes extended.

3. Inhale and lift the chin to the ceiling allowing the tummy to move towards the floor, concaving your back.

4. Exhale, round your back, tuck your chin, draw your navel in, and allow the head to face the mat.

5. Repeat 10 times.

2. Balasana – Child's Pose

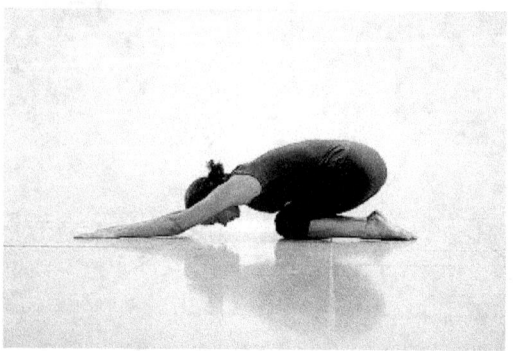

Yoga teachers recommend this pose to calm the wavering mind instantly. It massages your abdomen and circulatory system, promoting better flow of blood and oxygen, thus thwarting your anxiety.

How to do:

1. With the last exhalation in Cat-Cow Vinyasa, sit back on your heels, while folding the body forward, allowing the stomach to rest in between the knees.

2. Stretch the hands to your front and make a pillow by stacking the palms. Rest the forehead on the pillow.

3. Hold the posture, taking long, deep inhalations and exhalations for 10 breaths.

3. Adho Mukha Svanasana – Downward Facing Dog Pose

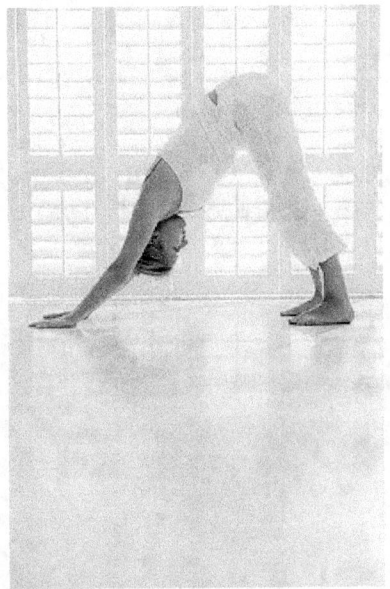

Stretch your body like a puppy and allow your nervous system to cool down with this intense stretching yoga posture. You are free to keep your knees bent, if you have a back or knee issue.

How to do:

1. With the final exhalation in Balasana, separate your hands and stack them under your shoulders.

2. Push your palms firmly into the mat and lift your body off from the heels to come into an inverted V posture.

3. Push your hips to the ceiling and heels to the mat.

4. Adjust the palms to stack your wrists under the shoulders.

5. Engage the core, thigh, and glutes and hold the posture for 5 long and deep breaths.

4. Malasana – Garland Pose – Complete Squat

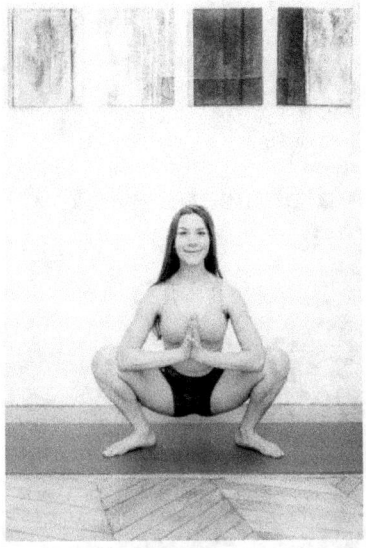

It is a calming pose that corrects your posture and allows the energy to flow through the spine. This, in turn, helps you relax and remain peaceful even during turbulent times.

How to do:

1. With the final exhalation in Downward Facing Dog pose, walk or jump in between the palms and squat down completely.

2. Separate your knees wider than the hips. Lengthen your torso and elongate your spine.

3. Join your hands at heart center, pushing the knees out with your elbows.

4. Close your eyes and hold the posture, breathing deeply for 5 deep breaths.

5. Paschimottanasana – Seated Forward Bending Pose

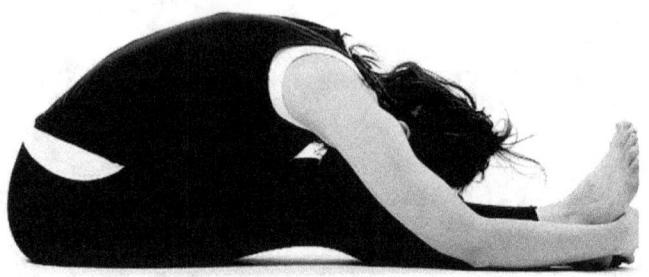

It calms the brain and helps in relieving stress and anxiety by stimulating better circulation to the brain.

How to do:

1. On the final exhalation in the Garland Pose, sit down on the mat and stretch your legs in front of you. Keep your feet flexed towards you.

2. Adjust your sitting bones and elongate the spine.

3. Inhale and sweep your hands over your head and lengthen the torso.

4. Exhale and fold forward from your hips, bringing the hands simultaneously with your body, and hold your feet, lengthening your spine forward. Do not round your back. If you are unable to hold your feet, hold wherever you are able to reach without rounding the spine.
5. Inhale, lift your chest, and look up. Exhale and fold forward completely, your tummy resting on the thighs and forehead on the shin.

5. Hold the posture for 5 deep breaths.

6. Parivrtta Sukhasana – Simple Seated Twist

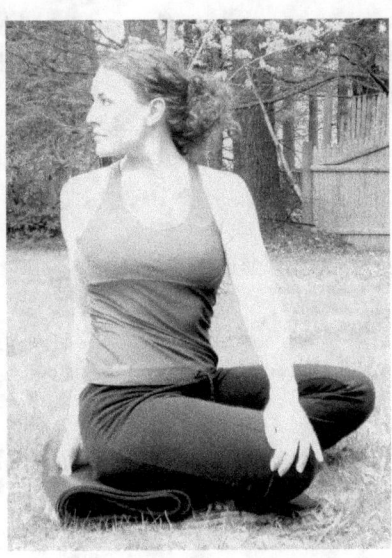

All twists help in detoxification. And, as the levels of toxins start diminishing, your circulation improves and you will become calmer and more peaceful.

How to do:

1. After you complete the fifth round of breathing in Pashimottanasana, inhale and straighten your torso.

2. Sit in cross-legged posture, keeping the spine erect.

3. Inhale and place your right palm on the left knee and allow the fingertips of left palm to rest behind you.

4. Exhale and twist to your right.

5. Suspend your breath and hold the posture, looking over your shoulders for a count of 10.

6. Inhale and come back to the center. Exhale and release the hands.

7. Repeat the same with the other side.

8. Repeat the twists three times.

7. Viparita Karani – Legs Up The Wall Pose

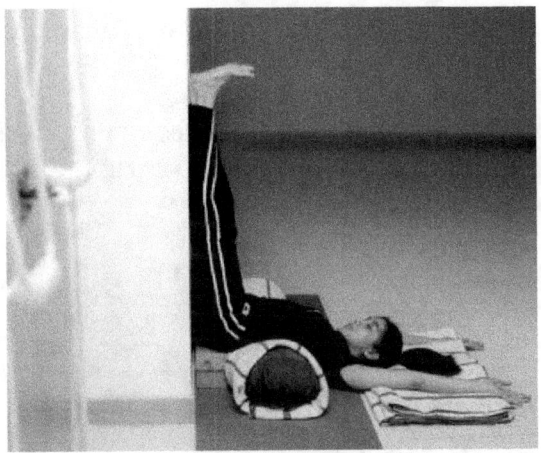

It is a gentler version of Sarvangasana, or the Shoulder Stand. An inversion posture, it is known to help you relax and unwind.

How to do:

1. Untwist your torso with the final exhalation and come to the center.

2. Sit against a wall, the left side of your body aligned along the wall. Bend your knees and rest it on your chest.

3. As you exhale, recline on the mat, resting the feet on the wall, keeping the knees bent.

4. Support your body with the elbows. Inhale and as your exhale, relax your lower back and stretch the arms over your head.

5. Hold the posture, breathing deeply, for 10 deep breaths.

6. To come out the pose, rest your knees on your chest and roll to your right and sit upright.

8. Matsyasana – Fish Pose

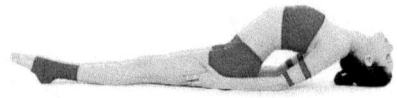

It is practiced as the counter pose to inversions. It stimulates the flow of blood into the endocrine system, stimulating the release of relaxation hormones.

How to do:

1. Recline on the mat, stretching your legs out, and resting the palms under your buttocks.

2. Inhale, lift your head up.

3. As you exhale, rest the crown of the head on the mat, lifting the chest up towards the ceiling. Keep the hips on the mat.

4. Hold the posture for 10 deep breaths.

5. Inhale, lift your head off the mat, look to the front, and place the back of the head on the mat.

9. Supta Baddha Konasana – Reclining Butterfly Pose

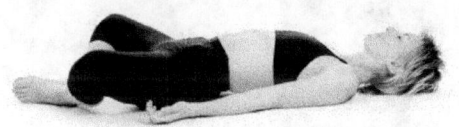

It is a restorative yoga pose that is used for meditation as well. It allows you to restore that natural state of inner calmness and peace.

How to do:

1. After you come out of Matsyasana, bend your knees outward to join the soles of the feet. You could keep a cushion to support your back.

2. Let your hands rest on either sides of the body, palms facing up.

3. Close your eyes and relax in the posture for 10 deep breaths.

4. Inhale, stretch out the legs and hands. Exhale and roll to your right.

5. Inhale and sit up in a seated posture of your choice and prepare yourself for the meditation.

10 Minute Meditation

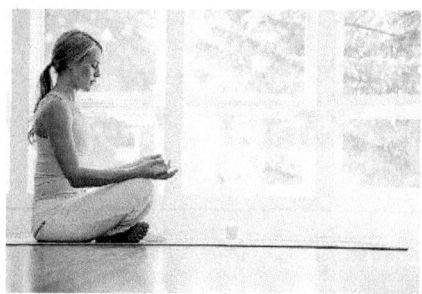

Studies reveal that spending a few minutes in meditation could help in calming your mind, bringing with it oodles of abundance. It restores your inner peace and calm. You can set your timer for 10 minutes to help you acquaint with the practice.

How to do:

1. Sit down in a comfortable seated poition, keeping your spine elongated. You can rest your back against your wall so that you will not be compromising on your spine.

2. Close your eyes and rest your hands on your knees.

3. Take long inhalations and exhalations and allow your body to calm down.

4. Focus on your breath.

5. Notice how your body moves with each breath.

6. Observe your shoulders, chest, rib cage, and abdomen rising and falling with inhalations and exhalations.

7. Make no conscious efforts to control your breath.

8. If your mind wanders, just return your focus to your breathing.

9. Practice this till your timer goes off.

10.

Once you are able to watch your thoughts and breath without judging, you will be able to calm your mind. Regular practice of these postures,

breathing technique, and meditation will surely
gift you the potential to stay calm even when
the tide is high.

Chapter 5

30 Minutes to Boost Your Confidence & Esteem

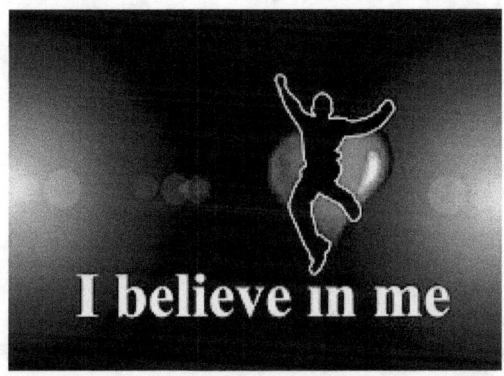

Low levels of self-esteem and self-confidence arise due to a wide array of external and internal factors. Negative self-talk, lack of proper support from the family and friends, constant admonishing, lack of proper education, growing up in a co-dependent family, unfair comparisons, and having conflicting and disapproving authority figures are some of the root causes of these conditions.

However, on an energetic level, reputed yoga gurus tell us that an underactive Solar Plexus is the root cause of low self-esteem. Balancing this Chakra or energy center that is located just behind your navel is essential to restore your power.

The sequence outlined below focuses on activating the Solar Plexus, thereby working on your inner self to boost your levels of confidence and esteem.

Warm Up With Breathing

There are various breathing techniques yoga teachers use to help a practitioner boost his/her self-esteem levels. One of the most commonly used breathing practice is the **bee breathing**, which is also known as *Brahmari Pranayama.*

This breathing technique elevates your mood and eliminates all self-pity, clearing the way for improved confidence and esteem. An energy boosting Pranayama, it improves circulation and heals anxiety.

How to do:

1. Sit in a comfortable seated posture on the mat, keeping the spine erect.

2. Rest the tips of your index fingers slightly on the cartilages of respective ears.

3. Take a slow, deep inhalation.

4. As you exhale, press the cartilages with a mild pressure while humming like a bee.

5. Repeat the breathing technique for 5 minutes.

20 Minute Self- Esteem And Self-Confidence Boosters

1. Tadasana – Mountain Pose

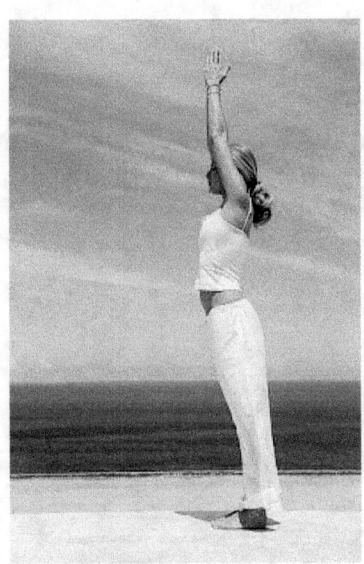

The body gets an entire stretch, stimulating the circulation and uplifting the mood, esteem, and confidence. This is a variation of the posture wherein your heels are off the floor and you are balancing on your toe tips.

How to do:

1. Stand on the mat, feet touching each other, spine erect, and arms resting alongside the body.

2. Inhale and sweep your hands over your head. Join your palms or interlock your fingers, palms facing the Crown of your head.

3. Exhale and lift the heels and come on your toe tips.

4. Hold the posture, engaging the core and squeezing the buttocks, breathing deeply for one minute.

2. Vrkshasana – Tree Pose

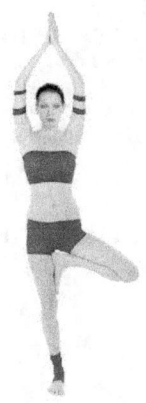

Regain and restore your natural state of balance and redefine your esteem and confidence levels with this Tree Pose.

How to do:

1. With the final exhalation in Tadasana stretch, release the feet back on the mat.

2. Inhale, bend your right knee and rest the sole of the right foot on the left inner thighs.

3. Keep your hips squared to the front of the mat and spine erect.

4. Exhale and as you inhale, sweep your hands over your head and join your palms.

5. Focus at a point in front of you and hold the posture for one minute, breathing deeply.

6. With the final exhalation, release your right leg.

7. Repeat the same with the other leg for one minute.

Tips

- Place your hands at your hips if you are finding it difficult to balance.

- You can also take the support of the wall till you get accustomed to the practice.

3. Virabhadrasana I – Warrior I Pose

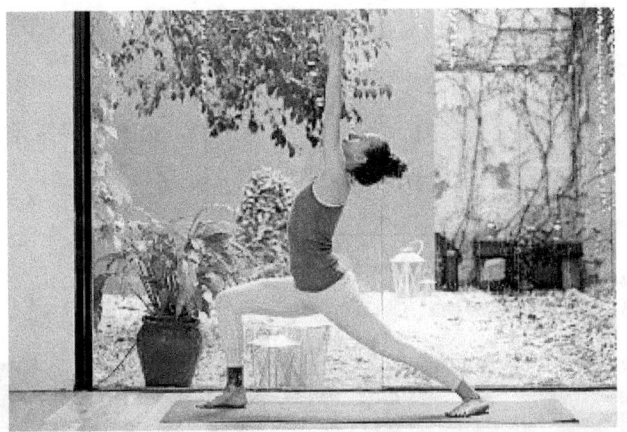

Build your courage and boost your self-assurance like a warrior by including this simple posture in your daily routine.

How to do:

1. Exhale and release the left leg.

2. Inhale and extend the left leg back, bending the right knee and stacking it over the right ankle.

3. Exhale and sink your hips down, while keeping it squared. Engage your core, buttocks, and thighs.

4. Inhale and sweep your arms over your head and join the palms.

5. Exhale and gaze at the fingertips.

6. Hold the posture, breathing deeply, for one minute.

7. With the final exhalation, lower the hands and join the feet.

8. Repeat the same with the other side for one minute.

4. Virabhadrasana II – Warrior II Pose

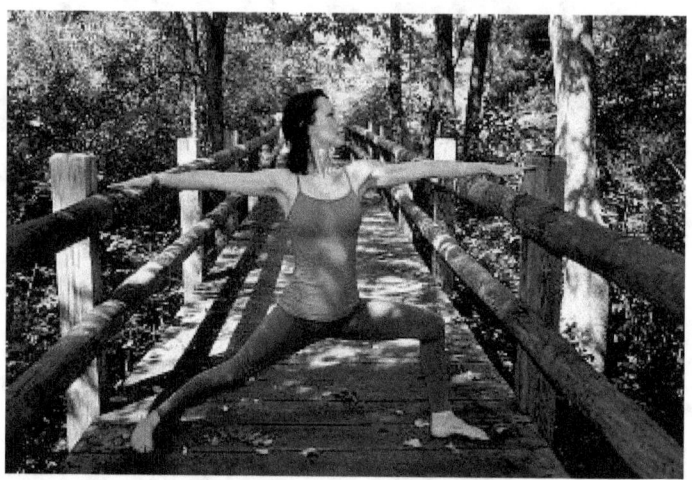

This pose is also quite often practiced in a self-esteem and confidence building yoga session. Along with stretching and stimulating your spine, it helps in opening up your navel and heart chakras.

How to do:

1. With the final exhalation in Warrior I, release your hands.

2. Inhale and turn your hip towards your right.

3. Place your right foot firmly on the mat, turning it slightly towards your left foot.

4. Exhale and extend your hands at shoulder level allowing your left hand to come in front of you and right hand to your back.

5. Engaging the glutes, core, and quadriceps, sink your hips lower.

6. Fix your gaze at the left fingertips.

7. Hold the pose, breathing deeply, for one minute.

8. Exhale, release the hands, and join the feet.

9. Repeat the same on the other side.

5. Utkata Konasana – Goddess Pose

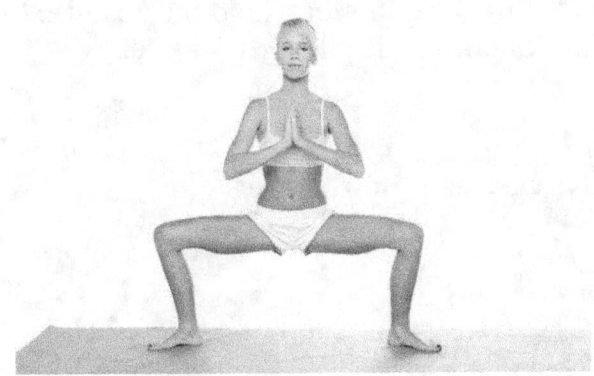

Awaken the strength of your Inner self and enhance your poise and grace with this fabulous hip opener.

How to do:

1. From Warrior II, as you complete the final exhalation, join your feet.

2. Inhale and separate your feet, angling it away from the body, making a 45 degree angle with the legs.

3. Exhale and as you inhale, bend the knees in such a way that thighs are parallel to the mat.

4. Exhale and sink the tailbone until it is aligned with the knees. Keep your spine and head aligned.

5. Join your palms at heart center, keeping the elbows parallel to the mat.

6. Engaging the core, hold the posture, breathing deeply for 1 minute.

6. Navasana – Boat Pose

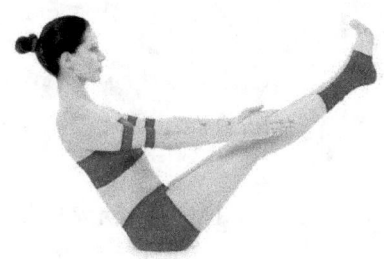

This posture works wonderfully on the core, toning it and activating your self-esteem center. Studies suggest that people who practice this posture regularly hardly experience bouts of low confidence and self-esteem.

How to do:

1. With the final exhalation in Goddess Pose, sit down on the mat, extending the legs in front of you.

2. Lengthen and align your spine, neck, and head. Flex your feet towards the body.

3. Inhale and elongate your torso.

4. Exhale and lean back slightly, engaging the core. Simultaneously, lift the legs off

the floor, balancing your body on your sit bones. Your torso and legs should be angled at 45 degrees.

5. Lift the hands and stretch it out to the front, allowing it to come parallel to the legs. Alternatively, you can rest the fingertips on the mat.

6. Inhale and bring the navel close to the spine.

7. Breathing deeply, hold the posture for 1 minute.

7. Purvottanasana – Upward Facing Plank Pose

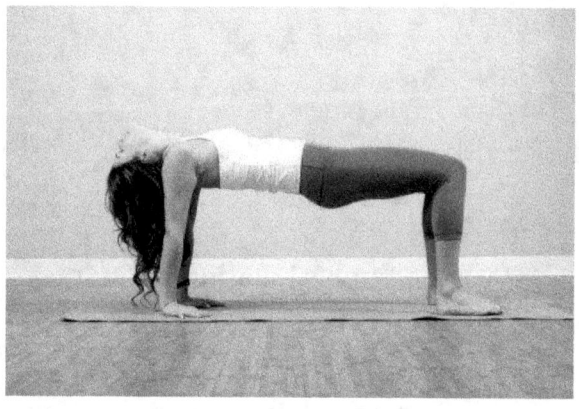

This posture is the counter-pose to Boat Pose and sets your confidence and esteem levels soaring.

How to do:

1. With a final exhale in Navasana, rest the feet on the mat, knees bent and kept at hip distance.

2. Place the palms behind your hips, fingers pointing towards you.

3. Stack your shoulders and wrists.

4. Inhale and as you exhale, press the palms and feet into the mat and lift the torso up, allowing the hips to come parallel to the mat.

5. Fix your gaze on the ceiling and breathing deeply, hold the posture for 1 minute.

6. Inhale and as you exhale, release the posture and stretch out your legs.

This completes one round of the sequence. Repeat the sequence one more time to complete you 20 minute self-esteem boosting daily yoga routine.

Wind up with Makarasana

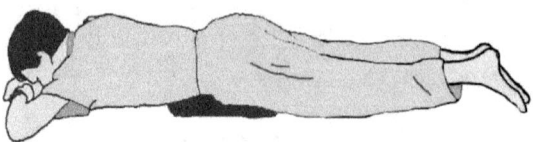

This is a restorative and relaxing yoga posture that helps you learn to surrender yourself to the Inner Self and trust yourself. Self-trust is the key to enhancing your self-esteem.

How to do:

1. Once you complete the second round of the sequence, lie down on your tummy.

2. Fold the hands in front of you, making a cushion with the same. Rest the forehead on this cushion.

3. Rest the toes in a relaxed way.

4. Close your eyes and breathing deeply, relax and surrender.

5. Hold the posture for 5 minutes.

6. To come out, stretch out your hands in front of you.

7. Roll to your right and sit upright in any seated posture of your choice. Keep your eyes closed.

8. Rub the palms to generate heat. Place it on your eyes. Gently open your eyes.

Yoga alone might be not be useful in restoring your confidence and esteem levels. Think positive and start loving yourself. Learn to accept yourself unconditionally. Stop comparing yourself with others. You can also use various affirmations to boost your self-esteem. Here is a sample.

"I love and accept myself unconditionally. I approve of myself and feel great about myself. I have high self esteem as I respect myself."

Keep chanting these affirmations as you practice the postures and breathing techniques. Slowly, you will feel the difference!

Chapter 6

How to master your practice?

"Do your practice and all is coming." ~
Sri K Patthabi Jois

You need to practice to experience the benefits.
And, there is no shortcuts to master your
practice than practice the routines regularly
and dedicatedly. Here are some tips you could
follow to master the sequences:

1. Always practice on an empty stomach.
That is why yoga teachers advise you to indulge
in a yoga session early in the morning. If you
are practicing otherwise, make sure you do not
have any solid food for 3 hours at least. Refrain
from drinking liquids at least one hour before
your session.'

2. Wear comfortable clothing.

3. Practice around the same time daily.

4. Practice in the same place to boost the levels of your benefits.

5. Listen to your body. Be gentle with it.

6. Play some soothing music that would boost your morale.

7. Do not forget to breathe.

Last, but not the least, enjoy and savor the experience. That is what finally counts. A practice that is done whole-heartedly yields quicker and more effective results.

"It's not what we do once in a while that shapes our lives. It's what we do consistently," Goes the words of Anthony Robbins.

So start practicing and stay consistent! You will see the results very soon!

Conclusion

"Habits allow us to not think about what we're doing . . . giving us the illusion of ease. When we are under the illusion of ease, not thinking about what we're doing. Breathing the same old way, moving the same old way, thinking the same old way we check out of the present, out of happiness itself, " says Alex Levin.

It is now time to break your habits. Step out of your comfort zone and challenge yourself. Do not fear the change. Welcome it with all your heart, unconditionally. Everything happens for your higher good, to help you grow and blossom.

According to Petri Räisänen, "When you listen to yourself, everything comes naturally. It comes from inside, like a kind of will to do something. Try to be sensitive. That is yoga."

Learn to listen to your body and mind with these simple sequences and let the results come naturally…

Happy yogaying...

Namaste!

BEFORE YOU GO

If you liked this book you may like these other books from Mark Thomas

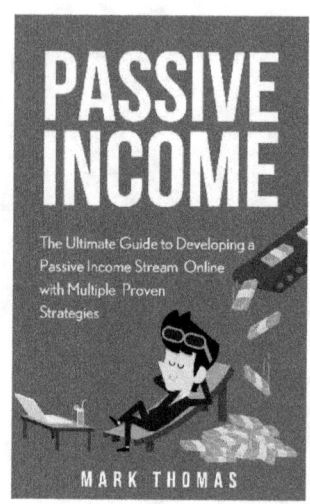

>>Check out more books by Mark Thomas<<

Free Gift

As Promised Here Is Your Guide To
Creating More Hours In Your Day:
Discover How To Fit 48 Hours Of Work
In A Day

GET YOUR COPY

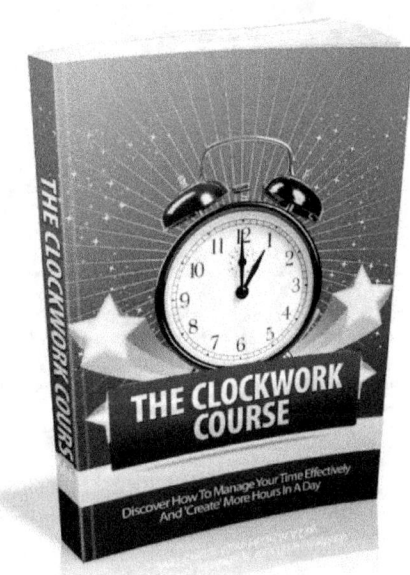

LEARN HOW TO GET MORE DONE IN A DAY

Do you feel stuck, stressed, and pissed because you aren't able to get all of your most important tasks done in a day? Perhaps this book can be the answer to your struggles. Learn the ways to manage your time to get more things done in a day and free up time do things you enjoy in life. Procrastination and Distractions are the biggest enemy of time management. This book will teach you the exact strategies to conquer procratinsation.

If You Want Free Best Selling Kindle Books Delivered Straight To Your Inbox

JOIN OUR FREE KINDLE BOOK CLUB!

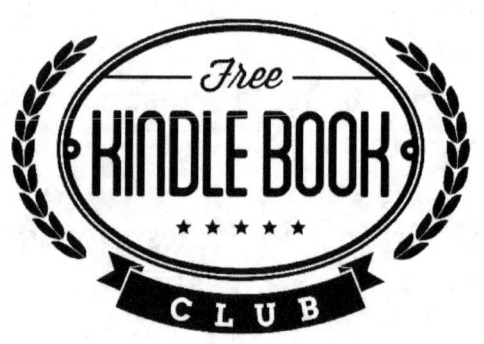

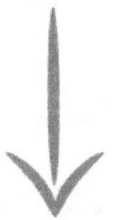

<u>CLICK HERE</u>

Chapter One – The Money Mindset

Before you even begin to think about making over ten thousand dollars in a month in just ninety days, you have to know what the proper mindset is in order to achieve that goal. You see, your mindset is extremely important to what you want to achieve. If you tell yourself

you can't do something, then you won't be able

to achieve it! So let's explore how you can have the proper money mindset in order to get rich!

First, let's take a look at an example of

someone who has a money mindset and

someone who doesn't. We'll take a look at two

handymen. Handyman one, let's call him George, walks into a home and he is approached by the homeowner. The homeowner tells him or her they want crown molding put in their upstairs bathroom. George affably agrees it will make the appearance of

their home nicer, but that's it.

Now, the second handyman's name is Josh. Josh walks into the home and he approaches the homeowner who tells him about wanting the crown molding. Josh also agrees it will look nicer, but he also goes on to explain how the crown molding will improve the value of the home over the long run.

Do you see the difference? George just wanted to make the home look better for aesthetic purpose only, but Josh saw the *value* in putting the crown molding in from an investment standpoint.

Being able to see the value in something is the money mindset. There are numerous other aspects to the money mindset, so let's take a look at them.

#1 Mindful of the Long-Term

There are many people out there who are looking to make money fast, but they rarely ever make a lot of it because of greed. Their first mindset is to think about what's in it for them. Rather, they should be thinking about how they can add as much value to someone else first. For example, it's like building credits with someone or an organization over the long-term. You might never need to use those credits, but if you do, help is returned in abundance. Don't allow your short-term greed destroy your long-term wealth.

#2 You Deserve Only What You've Earned

There is no room for an attitude of entitlement for someone when they have a money mindset.

Don't expect to get to the corner office without paying your dues. At sixty-three years old, the man who put up the crown moldings is a great example of someone who doesn't expect something. He comes in with a good attitude to his job, does it well, cleans up, and leaves.

#3 You Believe You Deserve to be Wealthy

Money is out there for anyone to get their hands on. Once you believe you deserve to have that money, you'll subconsciously change your actions to make it happen. Stop feeling guilty about earning six figures in a year. There are people out there who earn seven and drive their companies into the ground to do it! Your mindset should not be 'why me' but 'why *not* me'? With the belief that you deserve to be wealthy too, your income will soar!

#4 You Ask Yourself What the Value of The Product or Service is Before You Spend a Dollar

People who have the money mindset are very value aware. Since they realize how hard it is to make money, they are much more careful about spending their money than the average person. They have to ask whether one dollar spent might return that dollar in the future. They are on the lookout for great deals and tend not to feel buyer's remorse because they purchase things that have a greater value than what they paid.

#5 You're Always Looking for Synergies and Leverage

When you go out to play tennis with people at a club or you're hanging out with some new friends, get excited! There could be synergies involved with those people. Not only are you having a good time with those people, but you are parlaying your relationship right into an excellent business opportunity. A website is an excellent example of leveraging assets to earn more. Besides earning advertising money, you can earn money by selling products and services. Your website can also serve as an online resume PR hub if you want to do more public works. If you haven't started a website, you really ought to!

#6 You Realize a Dollar Spent Today Could Grow To Much More In The Future

People who have the money mindset are naturally frugal. They despise letting go of too much money because they've already figured out what they spent today might have turned into if they had saved and invested at a ten percent rate of return over the following five to thirty years. Compound growth anchors money mindset people into spending less than they have earned. With an aggressive savings rate, you'll be surprised with just how much you could accumulate in a 401k in ten years.

#7 You're All About Tax Optimization

It's imperative to think about how much you have to earn before purchasing a particular item due to taxes. A car that costs $21,000 requires you to actually earn $30,000 in gross income. In terms of making money, someone who has a money mindset will look to reduce their taxes by figuring out the most tax friendly way they can make money passively, such as dividends. They also look to synergize their expenses if they are a freelancer or small business. There's no reason to do a company offsite in North Dakota if you can do one in Kauai. Figuring out how to pay little or no taxes becomes a hobby for someone with a money mindset.

#8 You Believe Excuses are No Excuse

You're either going to make it happen or you're going to fail. Failure is just fine; just don't make excuses and not do something about it. Figure out the reasons why you failed and then try again until you succeed. You need to believe you deserve only what you've earned, you take ownership for your failures and you most past them. Excuses are for those who blame the world for their shortcomings rather than themselves. The more excuses you use, the less you believe you are able to make things happen on your own.

#9 You Never Fail Due to a Lack of Effort

You can fail because your competition is incredibly talented, there was bad timing, or a natural disaster happened, but you will never fail due to a lack of doing your best. There are many people out there who say they are going to make a living writing or freelance programming, but most of them won't even send a draft of what they're writing to someone else for feedback. They don't want to put in the time to make the money.

#10 You Execute Solutions

Recognizing a problem or coming up with an idea is one thing. Coming up with the solution is more important. There are so many people out there who like to point out injustices or complain about something, but none of them doing anything about the situation. Someone with the money mindset will find a way to get it done and make it better.

If you read through this chapter and you believe you don't have the money mindset, don't despair! Anyone can develop the money mindset. The first step is to know you're worth it and believing that you deserve to be wealthy.

If you put in the effort, there is no reason you can't be enjoying that passive income flow, too.

Now that you know what the money mindset is and you know where you have to change in order to become wealthy with passive income let's look at the amazing ways you can make ten thousand dollars in a month in just ninety days!

>>Check out more books by Mark Thomas<<

Finally, if you enjoyed this book, then I'd like to ask you for a favor, would you be kind enough to leave a review for this book on Amazon? It'd be greatly appreciated!

Thank you and good luck! ☺

www.ingramcontent.com/pod-product-compliance
Lightning Source LLC
Chambersburg PA
CBHW062016280526
45787CB00005B/2126

* 9 7 8 1 5 3 3 2 7 6 3 6 0 *